THE ULTIMATE SIRTFOOD DIET BOOK #2020

Easy and Healthy Weight Loss Recipes for Every Day incl. 28 Days Weight Loss Challenge

MATTHEW K. WILLIAMS

ISBN- 9798656867948

TABLE OF CONTENTS

The Sirtfood Diet

Have you ever heard of a diet which includes red wine, coffee, and even chocolate? An alimentary regimen which allows you to eat your favourite food without counting calories nor fasting?

If this sounds a little bit too good to be true, then you should try the Sirtfood diet.

What Is the Sirtfood Diet?

The Sirtfood diet was created by two nutritionists, Glen Matten and Aiden Goggins, who were working in a famous gym in the UK. When studying this new alimentary regimen, they wanted to find the perfect balance between the maximum Sirtfood intake and calorie restriction.

When they finally felt ready, they tested the diet on several participants from a London gym. All the participants lost an average of 3 kg (about 7 lbs) just in the first 7 days, despite not controlling their calorie intake or increasing the levels of exercise. Besides, the majority of participants gained muscle, whereas it usually happens the opposite when dieting.

They then understood how impressive this diet was and they shared it with people by writing their book, "The Sirtfood Diet: The Revolutionary Plan for Health and Weight Loss".

Nowadays, several celebrities advocate that they lost weight thanks to this alimentary regimen, and many people are excited to try its benefits.

What Are Sirtfoods?

Sirtfoods are a group of nutrient-rich foods which are believed to be able to rejuvenate your body cells, activating your "skinny genes" (which are known as sirtuins). In other words, they work on our body in the same way as other fasting diets do, but with more benefits.

What Are the Best Sirtfoods Nutrients?

The best way to benefit from this diet is to eat lots of food that contain sirtuin-activating nutrients. The most common Sirtfood-rich ingredients that you should include in your daily food are:

- ✓ Dark chocolate (at least 85% cocoa)
- ✓ Citrus fruits
- ✓ Turmeric
- ✓ Parsley
- ✓ Kale
- ✓ Capers
- ✓ Blueberries
- ✓ Green tea
- ✓ Apples
- ✓ Red wine (only starting from phase 2 of your diet)

Is the Sirtfood Diet Healthy and Sustainable?

Sirtfoods are healthy for our body, and they have undeniable benefits for human beings as they are rich in anti-inflammatory and antioxidant properties.

On the other hand, you cannot expect that a handful of certain foods can automatically meet all the nutritional needs of your body. This is one of the main reasons why the Sirtfood diet is healthy and effective. This isn't a restrictive dietary regimen, where you must say goodbye to your favourite food.

All your need to do is to prefer certain ingredients while exercising and restricting your calorie intake.

The Sirtfood green juice, that you must drink up to three times per day, is also a perfect source of minerals and vitamins.

The Side Effects of the Sirtfood Diet

Before starting your diet, you must be aware of the importance of restricting your daily calorie intake, especially in the first two weeks of this alimentary regimen. Besides, you must be ready to drink the green juice and adopt this new lifestyle on a regular basis, and not just for one month.

At present, there are no significant side effects known when it comes to the Sirtfood diet. For this reason, it can be considered a safe lifestyle, although it is recommended to speak to your dietician or your doctor before starting any new diet.

The major side effect of this diet is hunger. Your body will need some time to adapt to a 1,000-1,500 calories regimen. Nevertheless, the green juice is rich in fibre, a nutrient that will help you feel full and thus make your transition to the Sirtfood diet easier.

Some people report some additional side effects during phase one, such as irritability and fatigue. These are all due to the calorie restriction and are very common to all diets of any sort.

As mentioned, it is always a good idea to speak with your doctor before changing your lifestyle. This also applies in case you have any concerns after a few days of Sirtfood diet, or if you wish to learn more about the benefits or side effects of this regimen for your body. If you suffer from certain conditions, seeking the advice of a medical professional is imperative and essential for your health.

Can I Exercise on a Sirtfood Diet?

Exercising is the best way to lose weight, live a healthy lifestyle, and feel better with our body.

If you wish to try the Sirtfood diet, you are not required to say goodbye to your gym or your favourite sport. Nevertheless, you should stop or reduce exercise at least during the phase one of your diet, which is when your calorie intake is drastically reduced. The best way to go through these first two weeks of your new lifestyle is to listen to your body, and remain focused on your goal. Don't forget to provide your metabolism with the adequate intake of protein and fibre, and you will soon be ready to rock the gym once again!

Once the Sirtfood diet becomes your new lifestyle, you can normally exercise. However, you should always try to consume protein after your workout. Luckily, there are several Sirtfood snacks which can help your body recover after an intense session in the gym.

If you believe that your fitness routine needs to be changed in accordance with your new diet, you should speak with a doctor or a personal trainer. Normally, the body needs a few weeks to get used to a new diet, and this may mean that you may feel more fatigued or hungry after your workouts.

Finding the perfect balance between your time at the gym and your new diet is very important, and it will be one of the essential milestones in your Sirtfood journey.

On the other hand, if you have never exercised, your new lifestyle can be the perfect opportunity to start doing it. This will boost your weight loss and your confidence in yourself!

Is the Sirtfood Diet Effective?

The Sirtfood Diet was developed by two nutritionists, which were working for an English private gym. Together, they realised how, by eating the right ingredients, one can easily lose weight by turning on their "skinny gene".

Of course, several scientists and nutritionists have questioned the Sirtfood Diet. Although there have been only a few long-term human studies to determine whether this dietary regimen has any significant health benefits, many people have reported good results after eating more Sirtfood ingredients for at least 4 weeks.

The authors of the diet themselves reported the positive results of their pilot study, which involved 39 participants from the fitness centre where the two nutritionists whre employed.

At the end of the first week of their "experiment", all participants lost an average of 3 kg (7 pounds). Besides, some of them managed to maintain or even gain muscle mass. This is extremely important since it is one of the most challenging results for all who decide to follow a diet to lose weight.

Why Is This Diet Effective?

It must be noted that, unlike other dietary regimens, the Sirtfood diet does not promise any immediate and long-lasting weight loss. To lose some weight, you are supposed to restrict your calorie intake to 1,000 calories for at least the first one or two weeks, and you must exercise. In other words, with this diet, you are genuinely losing weight, as your body is encouraged to use up its emergency energy stores (also known as glycogen), and burn more fat.

By restricting your daily number of calories, your body needs to use glycogen. Each molecule of glycogen needs about 3 molecules of water to be stored in your body. This means that, by using glycogen, you are also getting rid of excess water, which is one of the main causes of the so-called "water weight".

The majority of weight loss in the first week of any diet usually comes from water, muscle and glycogen. Only a small part derives from burning actual fat. This is the reason why it is essential to follow your diet for more than one week or one month.

In many cases, as soon as your calorie intake increases, your body will start replenishing its glycogen stores. This will cause your weight to come right back. Nevertheless, with the Sirtfood diet, you can enhance your "skinny gene", meaning that your body will be more prone to burning fat and, consequently, losing weight.

How to Take Advantage of Sirtuins?

The main aim of the Sirtfood diet is to activate your sirtuins and thus help your body burn more fat.

Research has shown that fasting and exercise are good ways to activate sirtuins. However, cutting calories usually leaves us feeling hungry and frustrated. This is one of the main reasons why the majority of diets don't work.

The best way to activate and enhance your sirtuins is to understand that different foods have different effects on our bodies. For example, plant-based ingredients are rich in compounds called polyphenols, which can make our life healthier.

Nevertheless, even polyphenols are all equal. In fact, certain polyphenols may be more effective than others in weight loss, and to achieve a better distribution of fat in our body.

The basis of Sirtfood diet is thus to exploit all the best sirtuin-activating nutrients, which have the ability to turn our "skinny gene" on. This diet is a revolutionary lifestyle which allows you to eat delicious foods while activating sirtuins and achieving a better body. Finally, a diet which doesn't involve only calorie counting or eating low-fat and low-carb ingredients.

How to Get Enough Sirts?

Of course, for this diet to work properly, you must ensure you get enough sirts in your daily diet.

One of the easiest ways to introduce more sirts in your diet is to stick to green vegetables. Even 10 g of parsley added to your main salad or meal can make a huge difference.

Besides, sirts are in many of the foods that we all normally eat and enjoy every day. This includes onions, olives, apples and even olive oil. In other words, once you balance your daily calorie intake, following the Sirtfood diet is easier than it may seem, and you won't have to prepare odd recipes to lose weights.

One of the best things about the Sirtfood diet is that it allows you to have red wine and chocolate, which are usually forbidden by other alimentary regimens. In fact, both chocolate and red wine contain resveratrol. Of course, they must be consumed in moderation.

Turmeric and oily fish, if eaten at least twice per week, will provide your sirtuins and your body with a significant boost.

Understanding the Sirtfood Diet

How Does the Sirtfood Diet Work?

Based on the guidelines set by the two nutritionists which created the diet, the regimen is split into two phrases:

1. **Phase 1**: the first 7 days are known as the "hyper success phase". This is when you must prefer a diet rich in Sirtfood ingredients, and reduce your calorie intake.

2. **Phase 2**: also known as "maintenance phase", this includes the following two weeks of your diet. This is the best moment to consolidate your weight loss, but you will not need to keep controlling your calorie intake.

Phase 1: The Hypersuccess Phase

The first phase of this diet lasts one week, and it is when you must be very motivated to kickstart your new lifestyle. It may not be easy to get used to your new diet, but you should follow all the guidelines so you will soon be able to enjoy all its benefits.

The first 3 days of your Sirtfood diet are the most critical. To ensure that your weight loss is successful, your calorie intake must be restricted to 1,000 calories. Most importantly, your diet must consist of 3 Sirtfood-rich green juices and 1 Sirtfood-rich meal. You are also allowed to eat 2 squares of dark chocolate.

In the following 4 days, you can increase your calorie intake to 1,500. Every day you can have 2 Sirtfood-rich green juices and 2 Sirtfood-rich meals.

During this first week of your diet, you are not allowed to drink any alcohol. Nevertheless, you must stay hydrated, and you can drink plenty of water, coffee and tea (especially green tea).

Phase 2: The Maintenance Phase

During this phase, you don't need to focus on calorie restriction.

Every day, you can have 3 Sirtfood-rich meals and 1 green juice. If you are still hungry, you can have one or two Sirtfood bite snacks.

You are allowed to drink red wine during this phase, but you shouldn't have more than 2 or 3 glasses per week. As usual, you can drink water, coffee and tea freely.

What Happens After the First Three Weeks?

It is important to understand that the Sirtfood diet must be intended as a lifestyle rather than a one-off diet. In other words, you are always encouraged to keep eating Sirtfood-rich ingredients, as well as drinking your daily green juice.

Of course, this doesn't mean that you must eat the same food every day. There are plenty of delicious recipes that you can make at home, even if cooking is not usually your cup of tea. In this book, you will find lots of ideas, hints and tips for following this diet. Besides, you will find a 28-day meal plan, which will help you go through your first month and get used to this new, healthier lifestyle.

The Best Sirtfood Ingredients

Buckwheat: An Essential Ingredient of the Sirtfood Diet

Buckwheat is one of the main ingredients of the Sirtfood diet. Doctors usually recommend this ingredient to those who wish to eat healthier food and lose weight, as it is gluten-free and full of essential nutrients.

If you have never tried buckwheat, you may be worried it does not taste good or it may be difficult to cook. However, if you have already tried quinoa or any other grain, you will immediately like buckwheat as well!

What is Buckwheat?

Buckwheat is an ancient grain, which has been eaten in Eastern Europe and Asian for centuries. Although it is now becoming increasingly popular due to its health benefits, several people all around the world have been eating it for decades!

However, it must be noted that buckwheat is a fruit seed related to sorrel and rhubarb, rather than a cereal grain. Sometimes, because of its amount of complex carbs, it is still referred to as a pseudo-cereal, although it is completely different from quinoa and other similar ingredients.

In other words, despite its name, buckwheat is not related to wheat and has thus different nutritional values.

Why Should I Eat Buckwheat?

Buckwheat is a delicious and healthy alternative to rice, pasta, and couscous. This is one of the most versatile ingredients, it is naturally gluten-free and it is completely safe to eat.

This ingredient is particularly high in protein and fibre, as well as minerals. This includes magnesium, copper, and manganese. It is rich in vitamins B and, most importantly, it contains few calories and almost no fat.

If you need to eat food which is low on the glycaemic scale, then buckwheat is perfect for you. It is rich in nutrients and antioxidants, and it is often used as a "superfood".

Science has shown that a diet rich in buckwheat is linked to a lowered risk of developing high blood pressure and high cholesterol. As you can image, this food is also perfect to help weight loss and reduce food cravings.

How to Cook and Eat Buckwheat

You can find buckwheat in several shops, and it comes in different forms. For example, you can directly buy buckwheat seeds or, if you wish to integrate it into your diet, you can find buckwheat pasta or buckwheat noodles. If you like to express your creativity in the kitchen and you are always looking for new recipes, you can buy some buckwheat flour and use it to prepare delicious food yourself.

Some shops sell raw buckwheat groats, which can be toasted. In this case, they are referred to as kasha and have a nutty flavour, which makes them perfect for a quick and healthy snack.

To cook buckwheat, you can usually follow the packet instructions. As a general rule, you can just cook it for 10-15 minutes in boiling water, and then let it drain. Just like pasta and rice, you can make buckwheat al dente, or cook a little bit longer for a softer result.

If you are looking for something tastier, you can even toast buckwheat in the dry pan for a couple of minutes and then add boiling water, just like you would do to make risotto.

Bird's Eye Chilli: How to Spice Up Your Diet

One of the best Sirtfoods is Bird's Eye Chilli. It contains lots of healthy nutrients, such as Myricetin and Luteolin, which are responsible for activating sirtuins and helping your body burn more fat.

This food, often known as Thai chillies, is very common among different Sirtfood recipes. If you are not used to spicy food, you can still enjoy it. Try adding just half the chilli to your food every day, and you will soon fall in love with its taste!

Since Bird's Eye chilli is so important for this diet, we want to share more about the origin of this ingredient. It originates in the American. Christopher Columbus brought it back to Europe in the 25th century, and since then it has been regularly cultivated and eaten through the rest of the world.

Today, many people enjoy its pungent and particular heat. What you may not know is that, in nature, this characteristic helps the plant defeat against predators which try to feast on it.

At present, there are hundreds of varieties of Bird's Eye chilli, with different colours and taste. Most importantly, this ingredient is always suggested as part of several diets for losing weight. This is because of its chemical compound, which plays a key role in increasing your metabolism and your body temperature. As you can imagine, a faster metabolism translates into proper digestion, which makes it less likely for your body to accumulate fat.

Extra Virgin Olive Oil: Is It Good for the Sirtfood Diet?

Several diets do not include olive oil, as it is believed to have too many fats and calories. However, extra virgin oil contains the best sirtuin-activating nutrients, which are Hydroxytyrosol and Oleuropein.

You can boost your skinny gene immediately just by adding two tablespoons of extra virgin oil a day to your diet. It will also provide your body with a lot of antioxidants. These are essential for protecting and straightening your immune system, making it more resistant to infection.

Most importantly, research has shown that, as a part of a balanced diet, extra virgin oil can help prevent or even delay the onset of diabetes. It also contains a substance known as oleocanthal, which has important anti-inflammatory properties.

Last but not least, olive oil has a high quantity of monounsaturated fat, which can help prevent or slow down Alzheimer and other cognitive decline associated diseases.

Matcha Green Tea: The Powerful Sirtfood from japan

Matcha has been known and consumed in Japan since the 12th culture.

Differently from any other green tea, matcha originates from a plant known as Camelia synesis, which is native to China. The shrub of this plant produces several leaves, including those used to produce the Pu-erh and the green oolong teas.

Matcha can be enjoyed on its own or as an ingredient for delicious green smoothies and, of course, the Sirtfood green juice. Since it is usually sold as a powder, you can mix it with your flour or other ingredients to make desserts, cupcakes, and even ice cream.

How Does Matcha Taste?

Matcha is particularly healthy as its leaves are not heated nor processed. This allows them to keep all their natural nutrients and taste. This is also one of the reasons why matcha green tea has a bright green colour. The powder needs to be stirred in warm water or milk, usually with a bamboo brush.

Matcha tastes slightly like grass, although it also has a rich, almost buttery flavour. To make it even more delicious, it is recommended to stir in the powder with non-dairy milk alternatives. If you think it is too bitter, you can add a bit of stevia or vanilla extract.

The Benefits of Matcha

Many people wonder why doctors usually recommend drinking matcha rather than any other green tea. This is due to the superfood benefits of this rich, green powder.

For example, matcha contains some of the most powerful superfood and sirtuin-booster nutrients we know of. It is also rich in antioxidants. In particular, it contains an antioxidant known as EGCG, which is linked to a healthier and faster metabolism, as well as improved ageing.

Matcha is also rich in anti-inflammatory nutrients, and it can really give your body a boost of energy. In other words, you can drink matcha before or after working out or jogging, and you will immediately feel better.

Because of its properties, matcha green tea can raise your metabolism. This makes it even more effective than coffee, which means that it is surely a good help to achieve weight loss. If you don't like exercising, or you are looking for a way to feel better, matcha will still provide your body with significant amounts of L-theanine. This is one of the amino acids that can promote a good state of relaxation, making matcha green tea one of the most calming beverages.

All the Benefits of Medjool Dates

Medjool dates originated in the Middle East and North Africa. Nowadays, they are cultivated in several desert-like places around the world and consumed almost everywhere because of their juicy and sweet taste.

You can enjoy Medjool dates on their own as a Sirtfood snack, or as a part of a salad or a healthy dessert.

Because of their properties, Medjool are often referred to as the king of dates. Besides, they tend to be bigger than other sorts of dates, and usually more expensive. Because of their juicy flesh, they are more difficult to cultivate and are thus rarer.

How Do Medjool Dates Taste?

Medjool dates are particularly sweet, although they do not have many calories. They have a caramel-like taste, which resembles honey and cinnamon. If you allow them to ripen, they will taste even sweeter.

Besides, as many Middle Eastern recipes suggest, they can be enjoyed alongside other ingredients, such as bread, crackers or cheese. Alternatively, you can get rid of the pit and serve them stuffed with almonds, walnuts or honeycomb.

Nutritional Properties of Medjool Dates

Medjool dates are one of the main Sirtfood ingredients. They have only a few calories and they are rich in fibre, essential minerals, magnesium, manganese, copper and potassium. In other words, they are perfect to boost your sirtuin and encourage your body to burn fat.

Because of their taste and their nutritional value, they are a particularly good alternative to other caloric desserts. You can enjoy them as an after-lunch snack without feeling guilty.

SIRTFOOD HEALTHY DRINKS

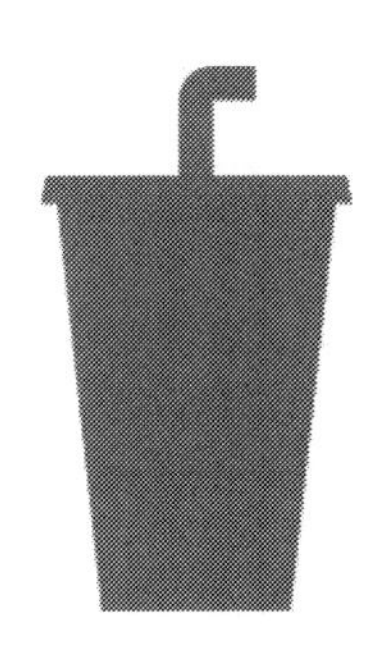

Sirtfood Diet Green Juice

***Difficulty:* Easy | *Calories:* 101 | *Servings:* 1**
***Fat:* 1 g | *Carbs:* 21 | *Protein:* 5 g**

Ingredients

- 75 g (2.6 oz.) kale
- 2 celery sticks
- 30 g (1 oz.) rocket
- ½ green apple
- 5 g parsley
- ½ tsp matcha green tea
- Ginger
- Juice of ½ lemon

Preparation

1. Put aside the matcha green tea and lemon, for now.
2. Juice all the ingredients together, until smooth.
3. Squeeze the juice of ½ lemon and stir well.
4. Pour the green juice into half of your glass or much, and add the matcha.
5. Stir in the matcha.
6. Add the rest of the juice and stir well.
7. Drink immediately or save for later. It can be stored for up to 3 days in the fridge.

Matcha with Vanilla

***Difficulty:* Easy | *Calories:* 12 | *Servings:* 1**
***Fat:* 0.2 g | *Carbs:* 1 g | *Protein:* 1 g**

Ingredients

- ½ vanilla pod
- ½ tsp matcha powder

Preparation

1. Pour warm water into a small bowl and whisk the vanilla seeds and the matcha powder together.
2. Discard the warm water and pour some boiling water.

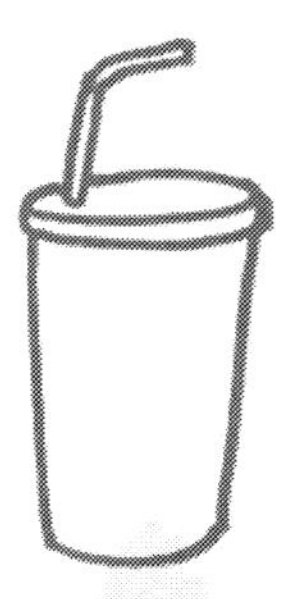

Turmeric Tea

Difficulty: Easy | Calories: 10 | Servings: 1
Fat: 0.5 g | Carbs: 1 g | Protein: 0.5 g

Ingredients

- 1 small orange
- 1 tbsp fresh grated ginger
- Honey or agave
- Lemon slices
- 3 tsp ground turmeric

Preparation

1. Mix the turmeric, ginger and orange zest in a teapot or jug.
2. Pour boiling water over the mixture.
3. Add some honey or agave and a slice of lemon.

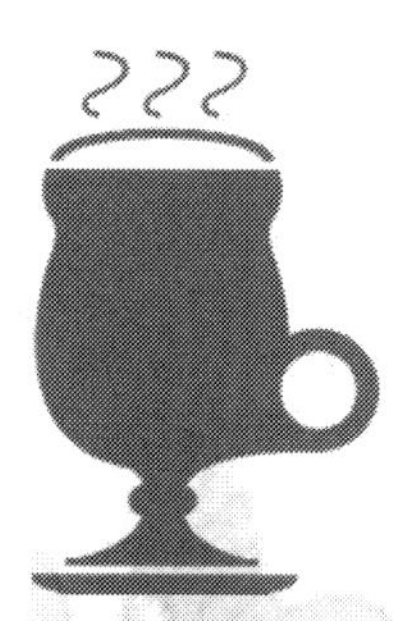

Sirtfood Quick & Easy Snacks

Often, following a diet to lose some weight means saying goodbye to snacking. Nevertheless, the Sirtfood diet allows you to indulge in your favourite snacks, especially if they are rich in sirtuin-boosters ingredients!

Let's take a look at the easiest, quickest and most delicious Sirtfood snack to make your diet easier.

1. Green Tea

Research has shown that green tea has a number of health benefits, and it is not surprising to find this beverage as one of the main Sirtfood snacks.

A cup of tea has 0 calories (unless you add some sugar) and will help you feel full and relaxed. You can drink as many cups of tea as you can per day, although you should stick to a couple and have it with no added sugar.

2. Dark Chocolate 85%

It may sound incredible, but you are allowed to have chocolate as a part of your diet and enjoy it without jeopardising your weight loss journey. 20 g of chocolate (which are about 6 squares) contains only 125 calories.

However, to be effective, you must choose 70% dark chocolate or, even better, 85%. Avoid milk or white chocolate, as they are rich in sugar and they are not very effective in boosting your sirtuins.

2. Cocoa

Just like chocolate, cocoa is a delicious and effective Sirtfood ingredient. 2 tsp of unsweetened cocoa only has 33 calories and can be mixed with boiling water to make a smooth and healthy instant hot chocolate.

3. Apples

They say that an apple a day keeps the doctor away. One apple has only 47 calories and it is a quick and easy after-lunch snack which will be 1 of your 5 Sirtfood a day. It is also the perfect way to keep sugar cravings away.

4. Red Grapes

Red grape is a very easy and delicious Sirtfood snack. It is also a low-calorie way to keep sugar cravings away. Always keep a portion of grapes in the fridge, or add them to your breakfast to feel full.

5. Blackberries and Blueberries

The average portion of blueberries and blackberries only has a few calories, and will immediately make any snack or breakfast more delicious. If you are looking for an easy way to boost your sirtuins, you should always keep them in your kitchen.

6. Pomegranate seeds

Pomegranate is one of the best fruits to boost your metabolism. It does thus not surprise If pomegranate seeds are effective in boosting our skinny gene.

7. Olives

Looking for a pre-dinner treat which will make you feel satisfied and not guilty? Then olives are the perfect solution for all your needs!

Sirtfood Delicious Recipes

Kale Omelette

***Difficulty:* Easy | *Calories:* 339 | *Servings:* 1**
***Fat:* 28.1 g | *Carbs:* 8.6 g | *Protein:* 15 g**

Ingredients

- 40 g (1.4 oz.) kale
- 1 small garlic clove
- ½ onion
- 3 eggs

Preparation

1. Shred the kale, slice the onion and mince the garlic.
2. Crack the eggs into a bowl, season with salt and pepper and whisk well.
3. Cook the kale and onion with a little bit of olive oil.
4. Add the garlic and cook for a few more minutes.
5. Add another tsp of olive oil and pour the egg mixture.

Easy One-Pot Vegan Paella

***Difficulty:* Challenging | *Calories:* 434 | *Servings:* 4**
***Fat:* 8 g | *Carbs:* 81 g | *Protein:* 9 g**

Ingredients

- 100 g (3.z oz.) peas
- 100 g (3.5 oz.) green beans
- 300 g (1 ½ cups) paella rice
- 1.2 l (5 cups) vegetable stock
- 1 onion
- 2 red or yellow bell peppers
- 2 lemons
- 2 tbsp olive oil
- 3 cloves garlic
- 3 tsp smoked paprika
- ½ tsp dried chilli flakes
- 3 medium tomatoes
- Saffron
- 2 tbsp chopped parsley for garnish

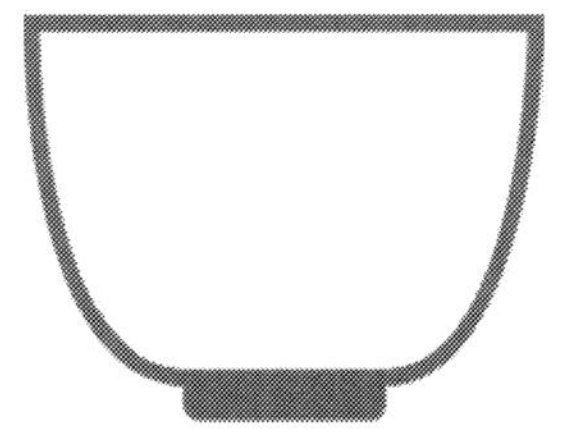

Preparation

1. Mix the saffron with the hot vegetable stock. Set aside.
2. Fry the onion in olive oil and leave to cook covered with a lid for 3 minutes.
3. Add the garlic, chilli and paprika. Stir well.
4. Then, add tomatoes, green beans, paella rice, bell peppers and the saffron vegetable stock. Leave to simmer for 15-20 minutes.
5. Add the peas and cook for 5-10 more minutes, or until the stock is completely absorbed.
6. Before serving, stir in the juice of 2 lemons and some chopped parsley.

Buckwheat with Mushrooms Salad

Difficulty: Easy | Calories: 168 | Servings: 1
Fat: 5 g | Carbs: 27 g | Protein: 7 g

Ingredients

- 100 g (3.5 oz) buckwheat
- 450 g (16 oz.) mushrooms
- 2 medium onion
- 3 tbsp butter
- 1 cup green onions
- Salt and pepper

Preparation

1. Cook buckwheat in boiling water for 20-25 minutes.
2. Melt the butter in a frying pan and cook the onions.
3. Add the mushrooms and leave to cook.
4. Combine the buckwheat with the mushroom texture and stir well.
5. Add some fresh green onions to garnish and season with salt and pepper before serving.

Kale Salad with Sun-dried Tomato Dressing

Difficulty: Easy | Calories: 623 | Servings: 4
Fat: 48 g | Carbs: 47 g | Protein: 7 g

Ingredients

- 100 g (3.5 oz.) fresh kale
- ¼ cup pine nuts
- 2 large avocados
- 2 medium apples

Dressing

- The juice of 2 oranges
- 125 ml (1 cup) water
- ½ cup chopped parsley
- 1 tsp pine nuts
- 6 sundried tomatoes
- 1 tbsp balsamic vinegar

Preparation

1. Let the tomatoes sit in a bowl under how water for 10 minutes, or until they soften.
2. In another bowl, mix the apples, pine nuts, kale and avocados together.
3. Drain the tomatoes and cut them into pieces.
4. Place all the ingredients in a food processor and blend until you get a smooth mixture.
5. Place the kale onto a serving plate and serve with the dressing.

Goat Cheese Salad with Walnut Dressing

Difficulty: Easy | Calories: 389 | Servings: 4
Fat: 29 g | Carbs: 31 g | Protein: 6 g

Ingredients

- 350 g (12 oz.) iceberg lettuce
- 170 g (6 oz.) cucumber
- 170 g (6 oz.) tomatoes
- 1 cup croutons or buckwheat to serve
- Goat cheese

Walnut dressing

- 100 g (3.5 oz.) walnuts
- 4 tbsp honey
- 6 tbsp extra virgin olive oil
- ¼ cup of water

Preparation

1. Cut all the vegetables into bite-size pieces and mix together into a bowl.
2. Add goat cheese and buckwheat or croutons.
3. Make the walnut dressing by processing the walnut until you get a smooth paste.
4. Add honey, olive oil and a bit of water to make the texture creamier.
5. Serve all the ingredients together.

Cashew Buckwheat Curry with Garlic Kale

Difficulty: Easy | Calories: 474 | Servings: 1
Fat: 31 g | Carbs: 45 g | Protein: 11 g

Ingredients

Cashew Curry

- 2 cloves garlic
- 1 onion
- 1 tsp turmeric
- 1 tbsp coconut sugar
- 1 tbsp grated fresh ginger
- 1 tsp smoked paprika
- 2 tbsp soy sauce
- 300 g (10.5 oz.) kale
- The juice of ½ lemon
- 200 g (7 oz.) buckwheat
- 100 g (3.5 oz.) cashews or peanuts

Garlic Kale

- 200 g (7 oz.) kale
- 2 cloves of garlic
- 1 tbsp oil
- 2 tsp maple syrup
- Salt and pepper

Preparation

1. Fry the chopped onion in coconut oil and add the grated ginger.
2. Add the buckwheat groats and cashews and toast them for a couple of minutes.
3. Add turmeric, smoked paprika, cumin, coriander and coconut sugar. Stir well.
4. Pour the soy sauce, coconut milk and sriracha (optional).
5. Stir in the chopped kale. Cover with water and leave to simmer for 20 minutes.
6. To make the garlic kale, fry garlic and kale in olive oil.
7. Add maple syrup and cook for 5 minutes.
8. Season with salt and pepper and serve with the curry.

Shaved Zucchini Salad with Walnuts

Difficulty: Easy | Calories: 247 | Servings: 4
Fat: 16 g | Carbs: 22 g | Protein: 8 g

Ingredients

- 1 zucchini
- ½ lemon
- 2 medium tomatoes
- 1 small onion
- 1 medium carrot
- ¼ cup walnuts
- 1 tbsp black sesame seeds
- Salt and lemon
- Fresh basil to garnish

Preparation

1. Peel the zucchini skin off.
2. Cut the tomatoes in halves or quarters.
3. Peel the carrot in thin slices.
4. Chop the walnuts.
5. Peel the onions and cut into pieces or thin rings.
6. Arrange all the vegetables onto a serving plate or in a salad bowl.
7. Season with salt and pepper, and lemon juice.
8. Add basil leaves and sesame seeds before serving.

Spicy Thai Pumpkin Soup with Ramen Noodles

Difficulty: Easy | Calories: 483 | Servings: 2
Fat: 41 g | Carbs: 28 g | Protein: 8 g

Ingredients

- 450 g (1 lb) pumpkin
- 1 tbsp Thai curry paste
- 1 medium onion
- 400 ml (13.5) tin coconut milk
- ½ mild chilli pepper (optional)
- 100 g (3.5 oz.) mushrooms
- Instant ramen noodles or buckwheat
- 1 lemon wedge
- Fresh parsley or coriander to garnish
- Salt and pepper

Preparation

1. Cook the diced onion and diced pumpkin in a pot with the Thai curry paste.
2. Pour the coconut milk and bring everything to a boil. Leave to simmer until the pumpkin is ready.
3. Meanwhile, cook the noodles or the buckwheat in boiling water.
4. Place the pumpkin in a food processor until you get a smooth texture.
5. Season with salt and pepper, and lemon juice.
6. Serve with your ramen or buckwheat, roasted mushrooms and fresh parsley.

Apple Chickpea Salad with Avocado Peanut Butter Dressing

***Difficulty:* Easy | *Calories:* 384 | *Servings:* 4**
***Fat:* 17 g | *Carbs:* 49 g | *Protein:* 12 g**

Ingredients

Apple Chickpea Salad

- 400 g (14 oz.) cooked chickpea
- 4 medium apples
- The juice of ½ lemon
- 2 tbsp extra virgin olive oil
- 1 tbsp paprika
- 2 celery stalks
- Fresh parsley to garnish

Avocado Peanut Butter Dressing

- The juice of ½ lemon
- 1 tbsp soy sauce
- 2 tbsp peanut butter
- 1 small ripe avocado
- 1 tbsp extra virgin olive oil

Preparation

1. Roast the chickpeas for 5 minutes in a frying pan.
2. Add paprika and stir well.
3. Combine chickpeas with roughly chopped parsley and lemon juice. Season with salt and pepper, if necessary.
4. Grate the apple and slice the celery. Throw both ingredients into a serving bowl.
5. Stir in the chickpeas.
6. To make the dressing, place all relevant ingredients in a food processor and combine until you get a smooth texture.
7. Serve the chickpeas with the dressing.

Buckwheat, Apple, Cranberry Avocado Salad

Difficulty: Easy | Calories: 268 | Servings: 4
Fat: 15 g | Carbs: 31 g | Protein: 35 g

Ingredients

- 1 medium Granny Smith apple
- 100 g (3.5 oz.) buckwheat groats
- 1 sliced ripe avocado
- Dried cranberries
- Baby arugula
- 1 clove garlic
- The juice of ½ lemon

Preparation

1. Bring the buckwheat groats to a boil and leave to simmer for 10 minutes.
2. Transfer the buckwheat to a serving bowl or place.
3. Add the apple, cut into matchsticks, and the remaining ingredients. Mix the salad well.
4. Season with lemon juice and olive oil. Additionally, you can use maple syrup or Dijon mustard.

Pasta with Spinach and Blue Cheese Sauce

Difficulty: Easy | Calories: 405 | Servings: 4
Fat: 17 g | Carbs: 50 g | Protein: 13 g

Ingredients

- 250 g (8.8 oz.) tagliatelle or your choice of pasta
- 150 ml (5.3 oz.) crème Fraiche
- 100 g (3.5 oz.) baby spinach
- 70 g (2.4 oz.) blue cheese
- 2 cloves garlic
- 1 tbsp olive oil
- Salt and pepper
- Chopped walnuts for garnish

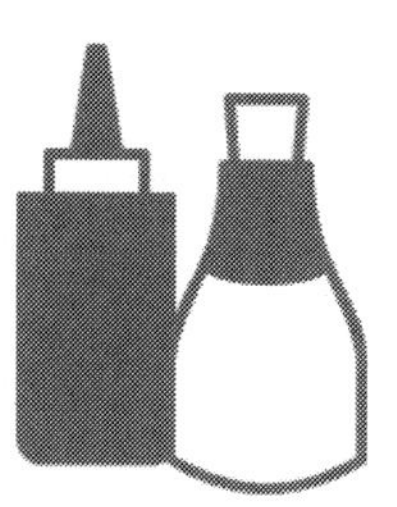

Preparation

1. Cook your pasta. When you drain it, don't forget to regain part of the cooking water.
2. Fry the garlic in olive oil for 2 minutes.
3. Add the garlic pan and crème fraiche.
4. Add the crumbled blue cheese. Season with salt and abundant black pepper.
5. Wait for the cheese to start melting, and then add the drained pasta and spinach.
6. Stir everything together and add a little of the pasta cooking water to make the blue cheese sauce creamier.
7. Garnish with chopped walnuts and serve hot.

Cheesy Buckwheat with Kale and Mushrooms

Difficulty: Easy | Calories: 365 | Servings: 6
Fat: 23 g | Carbs: 31 g | Protein: 45 g

Ingredients

- 100 g (3.5 oz.) buckwheat
- 55 g (2 oz.) Gruyere cheese
- 1 large egg
- Grated parmesan cheese
- 1 tbsp olive oil
- 225 g (8 oz.) mushrooms
- 170 g (6 oz.) kale
- 1 tbsp sliced garlic
- ½ diced onion
- Toasted walnuts for garnish
- Salt and pepper

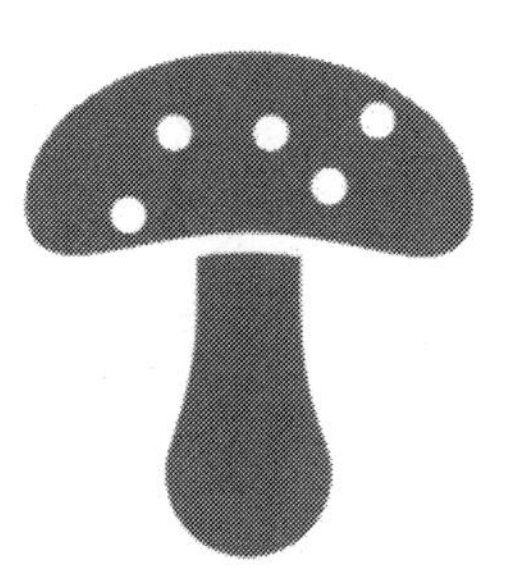

Preparation

1. Cook the buckwheat and combine it with the egg in a saucepan.
2. Bring to a boil and leave to simmer for 15 minutes.
3. Stir in both the Parmesan and Gruyere cheeses.
4. In another pan, heat the oil and fry the garlic, onion and mushrooms for 10 minutes.
5. Add kale and pepper and cook for 2 further minutes.
6. Mix the buckwheat mixture with the kale mixture.
7. Sprinkle with walnuts before serving.

Buckwheat and Beetroot Salad

Difficulty: Medium | Calories: 256 | Servings: 4
Fat: 16 g | Carbs: 15 g | Protein: 23 g

Ingredients

- 50 g (2 oz.) baby spinach
- ½ leek
- 3 large beetroot
- 100 g (3.5 oz.) roasted buckwheat
- 2 large garlic cloves
- 2 tbsp hazelnuts
- 1 tsp dried rosemary
- 3 tbsp olive oil
- 1 tbsp balsamic vinegar
- Salt and pepper
- Fresh parsley to serve

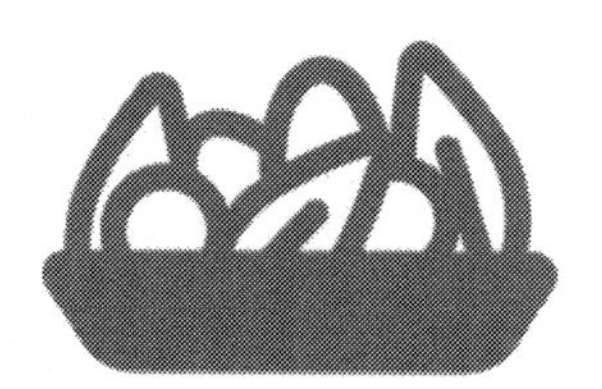

Preparation

1. Heat oven to 200 C (400 F).
2. Chop the beetroot into pieces.
3. Place beetroot in a bowl and season with olive oil, balsamic vinegar and pepper.
4. Combine dry rosemary and sea salt and process them with a pestle and mortar to get a fine powder. Use this rosemary salt to season the beetroot.
5. Cook the buckwheat.
6. Meanwhile, fry the leeks in olive oil with diced garlic.
7. Add mushrooms and keep cooking.
8. Season with salt, pepper and remaining balsamic vinegar.
9. Add spinach and then buckwheat.
10. Mix all the ingredients together.

One-Pot Harissa Chicken and Butternut Squash Pilaf

***Difficulty:* Medium | *Calories:* 623 | *Servings:* 4**
***Fat:* 15 g | *Carbs:* 85 g | *Protein:* 39 g**

Ingredients

- 500 g (1 lb) boneless chicken thigh fillets
- 600 ml (2 ½ cups) chicken stock
- 400 g (14 oz.) butternut squash
- 300 g (1 ½ cups) brown rice or buckwheat
- 1 red pepper
- 1 onion
- 2 tbsp olive oil
- 2 tbsp harissa paste
- 2 tbsp chopped parsley for garnish

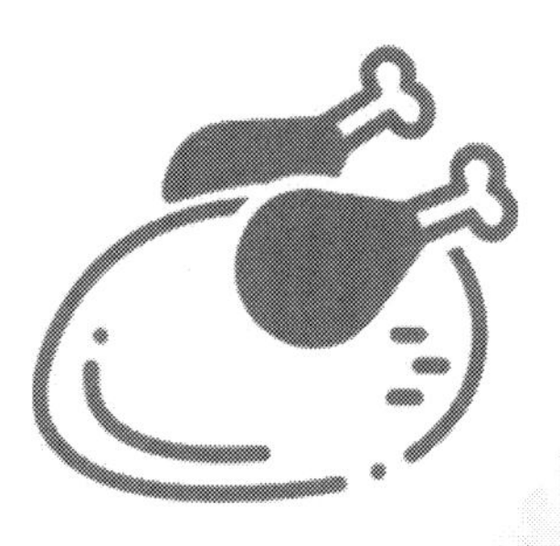

Preparation

1. Fry the peppers and onions in olive oil for 3 minutes.
2. Add the chicken thigh fillets and fry for 3-5 minutes.
3. Add the butternut squash, harissa pastes and stock.
4. Mix well and bring to the boil.
5. Cover with a lid and leave to simmer for 20 minutes.
6. Serve with parsley and brown rice or buckwheat.

Cider, Cream and Mustard Pork

Difficulty: Medium | Calories: 10 | Servings: 4
Fat: 18 g | Carbs: 6 g | Protein: 33 g

Ingredients

- 600 g (21 oz.) pork
- 100 ml (3.5 oz.) crème Fraiche
- 200 ml (7 oz.) cider
- 2 cloves garlic
- 1 onion
- 150 g (5.3 oz.) chestnut mushrooms
- 1 tbsp wholegrain mustard
- Salt and pepper
- Buckwheat and green vegetables to serve

Preparation

1. Cook the pork in olive oil for 2 minutes. Set aside and save its cooking juice.
2. Cook the sliced onion in oil, covered with the lid. After a few minutes, remove the lid and add the mushrooms and garlic.
3. Stir in the mustard and then add the pork back.
4. Add the cider and season with salt and pepper. Cook for 5 minutes.
5. Stir in the crème Fraiche and, when the pork is cooked through, serve with some buckwheat and your choice of green vegetables.

Yellow Split Pea and Spinach Dhal

Difficulty: Medium | Calories: 285 | Servings: 4
Fat: 5 g | Carbs: 47 g | Protein: 17 g

Ingredients

- 750 ml (26 oz.) vegetable stock
- 125 g (4.4 oz.) spinach
- 250 g (8.8 oz.) yellow split peas
- 2 cloves
- 3 cloves garlic
- 1 onion
- 1 tbsp olive oil
- 2 tbsp tomato puree
- 1 cinnamon stick
- 1 tsp cumin
- ½ tsp chilli flakes
- 1 tsp turmeric
- Grated ginger
- Buckwheat to serve

Preparation

1. Gook the diced onions in olive oil.
2. Add the garlic and ginger and leave to cook for 1 more minute.
3. Add the turmeric, cumin, cloves, chilli flakes and cinnamon. Cook for a couple more minutes.
4. Add the vegetable stock, tomato puree, and yellow split peas. Stir well and bring to the boil.
5. Cover with a lid and leave to simmer for 45 minutes.
6. When the dhal is ready, you can add the spinach. Cook for a few more minutes.
7. Serve with buckwheat or brown rice.

Lamb Jalfrezi

Difficulty: Medium | Calories: 354 | Servings: 4
Fat: 16 g | Carbs: 18 g | Protein: 33 g

Ingredients

- 600 g (21 oz.) diced lamb leg
- 1 red pepper
- 1 green pepper
- 400 g (14.1 oz.) tin chopped tomatoes
- 2 onions
- Grated ger
- 2 tsp coriander seeds
- 2 tsp cumin seeds
- 1 tsp chilli flakes
- 2 tsp turmeric
- 3 tsp garam masala
- 2 tsp fresh coriander
- 2 tbsp olive oil
- Buckwheat or cauliflower rice to serve

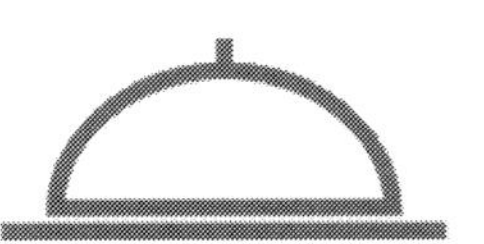

Preparation

1. Preheat oven to 180 C (400 F).
2. Cook the onion in a large saucepan with the olive oil for about 3 minutes.
3. Add cumin, coriander, chilli, ginger, garlic, turmeric and garam masala. Stir well and add a bit of water.
4. Add the lamb legs. After a few minutes, add the tomatoes.
5. Season with salt and pepper.
6. Bring it to the boil and then bake for 45 minutes.
7. Add the sliced peppers, stir well and leave to cook for another 45 minutes.
8. Serve with cauliflower rice or buckwheat.

Roast Beef Curry

Difficulty: Medium | Calories: 748 | Servings: 4
Fat: 59 g | Carbs: 26 g | Protein: 30 g

Ingredients

- 600 g (1 ¼ lbs) beef, chopped into pieces
- 1 red pepper
- 1 small sweet potato
- 2 onions
- 1 tin coconut milk
- 2 tbsp fresh coriander
- 2 tsp coriander
- 2 tsp cumin
- 2 tsp paprika
- 2 tsp turmeric
- 2 tsp garam masala
- 2 tsp tomato puree
- Salt and pepper
- Buckwheat to serve

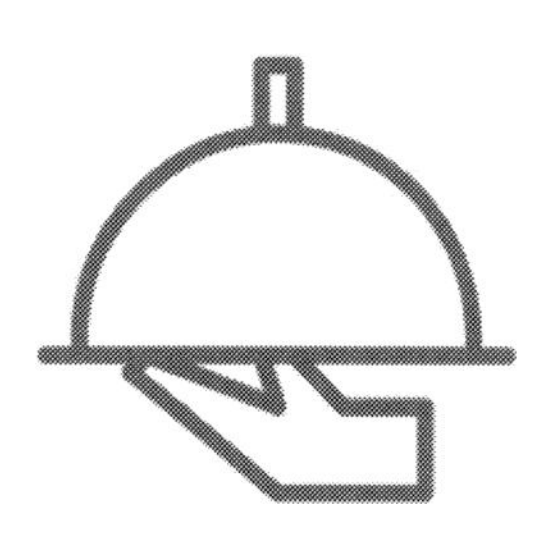

Preparation

1. Fry the onions in olive oil for 5 minutes.
2. Add ginger, chilli flakes, garlic and all the remaining spices. Cook for 1 minute. Add a bit of water if necessary.
3. Stir in the tomato puree and then add the coconut milk, red pepper and sweet potato.
4. Season with salt and pepper.
5. Cover with a lid and leave to simmer for 10 minutes.
6. Add the beef and keep cooking until the meat is ready.
7. Season with coriander leaves and the juice of half a lime before serving.

Spinach Style Red Wine, Borlotti Bean and Lamb Shank Casserole

Difficulty: Challenging | Calories: 413 | Servings: 4
Fat: 18 g | Carbs: 30 g | Protein: 27 g

Ingredients

- 400 g (14.1 oz.) tin chopped tomatoes
- 400 g (14 oz.) tin borlotti beans
- 150 ml (5.2 oz.) red wine
- 3 cloves garlic
- 1 medium carrot
- 1 medium onion
- 1 tbsp smoked paprika
- 1 tbsp cumin seeds
- 2 large lamb shanks
- 1 tbsp olive oil
- Fresh rosemary
- 2 tbsp parsley
- Buckwheat to serve
- Green vegetables to serve

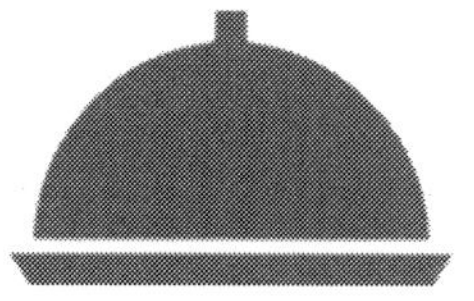

Preparation

1. Preheat oven to 150 C (350 F).
2. Season the lamb with salt and pepper, then put it in a large casserole dish greased with the oil. Leave it to brown on all sides.
3. Add the carrot and onion to the casserole.
4. Season with smoked paprika, rosemary, cumin, and garlic. Leave to cook for 5 minutes.
5. Add the red wine and leave to cook until it is reduced slightly.
6. Add the lamb shanks and tomatoes. Cover with a lid and bake for 45 minutes.
7. Turn the lamb and put back in the oven for another 40-45 minutes.
8. Add the drained borlotti beans and leave to cook for a final 30 minutes.
9. Serve with fresh parsley, your choice of green vegetables and buckwheat.

Pork Stroganoff

Difficulty: Medium | Calories: 568 | Servings: 4
Fat: 24 g | Carbs: 46 g | Protein: 39 g

Ingredients

- 200 g (1 cup) brown rice or buckwheat
- 150 ml (1/2 cup) sour cream
- 600 g (1 ¼ lb) pork loin steaks
- 100 g (3.5 oz.) chestnut mushrooms
- 2 tbsp chopped parsley
- 2 cloves garlic
- 1 tbsp olive oil
- 1 onion
- 3 tsp smoked paprika
- Salt and pepper
- Your choice of green vegetables to serve

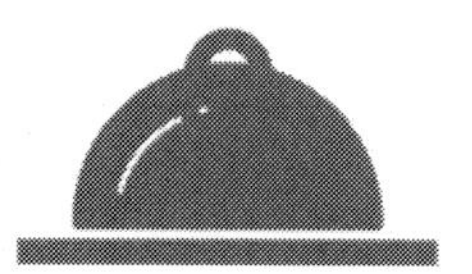

Preparation

1. Cook the brown rice or the buckwheat.
2. Fry the pork in olive oil for 5 minutes. Once ready, place the meat and its cooking juice onto a plate.
3. In the same pan, melt a bit of butter to fry the mushrooms and onions for 3 minutes.
4. When the mushrooms and onions are ready, season with paprika, garlic, salt and pepper. Stir in the pork with its juice and leave to simmer for 3-5 minutes.
5. Serve the pork and the sauce with your brown rice or buckwheat, and your choice of green vegetables.

Turkey Tikka Masala Meatballs with Bombay new Potatoes (with Raw Courgette Salad)

***Difficulty:* Challenging | *Calories:* 468 | *Servings:* 4**
***Fat:* 26 g | *Carbs:* 34 g | *Protein:* 30 g**

Ingredients

Turkey Meatball Tikka Masala

- 500 g (1 lb) turkey mince
- 200 ml (7 oz.) coconut milk
- 2 cloves garlic
- 1 tbsp + 1 tsp garam masala
- 1 tbsp olive oil
- 1 tsp paprika
- 1 tsp cumin
- ½ tsp chilli
- 1 red onion
- 1 tsp tomato puree
- Salt and pepper
- Fresh coriander
- Grated ginger

Bombay New Potatoes

- 400 g (14 oz.) new potatoes
- 6 small tomatoes
- 1 tsp cumin
- 2 tsp turmeric
- 1tsp mustard seeds
- 1 red onion
- Salt

Raw Courgette Salad

- 4 small tomatoes
- 1 large courgette
- 2 tbsp mint
- Juice of ½ lemon
- Salt and pepper

Preparation

1. Cook the potatoes in boiling water.
2. Meanwhile, prepare the courgette salad. You just need to mix all the ingredients in a bowl.
3. To make the meatballs, mix the turkey mince with 1 tsp garam masala and 2 cloves garlic. Season with salt and pepper.
4. Shape the turkey mixture into 20 meatballs and grill them for 10 minutes.
5. To make the masala sauce, you start by frying the sliced onions in olive oil.
6. Add more garam masala, garlic, paprika, cumin and chilli. Add some grated ginger and fry for 2 minutes.
7. Add the coconut milk to the masala sauce and the tomato puree. Season with salt, if needed. Leave to cook for 5 minutes.
8. Add the meatball to the sauce and leave to simmer for 10 minutes.
9. At this point, the potatoes should be ready. Fry them with some sliced onions in olive oil.

10. Add cumin, turmeric, potato and mustard seeds, and leave to cook for 2 minutes.

11. Serve everything together with some fresh coriander and the juice of ½ lemon. If you want, you can add additional seasonings, such as mango chutney or lime pickle.

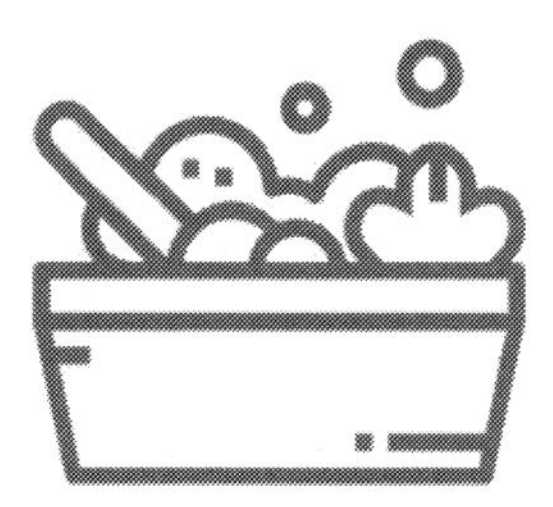

Sirtfood Diet: 28 Days Weight Loss Challenge

The Sirtfood Green Juice is an essential part of this diet. This means that, even when not mentioned, you should drink at least one or two glasses of this healthy juice every day. This will help your body burn calories and fat quicker, and you will soon see the difference in your weight!

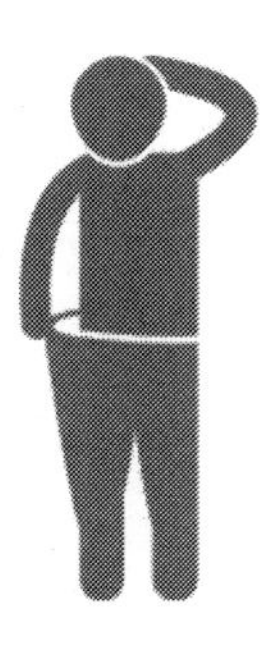

DAY 1

Breakfast: Green Juice (See page 24)

Lunch: Green Juice (See page 24)

Dinner: King Prawn Stir Fry with Buckwheat Noodles

Difficulty: Easy | Calories: 484 | Servings: 4

Fat: 10 g | Carbs: 65 g | Protein: 39 g

Ingredients

- 300 g (10.5 oz.) buckwheat noodles
- 1 red onion
- 100 g (3.5 oz.) kale
- 3 garlic cloves
- 500 g (17.5 oz.) king prawns
- 2 celery sticks
- 100 g (3.5 oz.) green beans
- 2 tbsp soy sauce
- 2 tbsp parsley
- ginger

Preparation

1. Cook the noodles, then drain and rinse in cold water.
2. Fry the celery and red onion in a wok.
3. Add the green beans and kale and cook for a couple of minutes.
4. Add garlic, ginger, chilli (optional) and prawns. Fry until the prawns are fully cooked.
5. Add the soy sauce and noodles and keep cooking for one more minute.
6. Sprinkle with parsley before serving.

DAY 2

Breakfast: Green Juice *(See page 24)*

Lunch: Chicken, Broccoli & Beetroot Salad with Avocado Pesto

Difficulty: Easy | Calories: 320 | Servings: 4

Fat: 18 g | Carbs: 8 g | Protein: 29 g

Ingredients

- 250 g (8.8 oz) broccoli florets
- 3 skinless chicken breasts
- 100 g (3.5 oz.) watercress
- 2 raw beetroots
- 1 red onion
- 2 tsp rapeseed oil
- Nigella seeds

Avocado Pesto

- 25 g (0.8 oz.) walnut halves
- Fresh basil
- 1 tbsp rapeseed oil
- ½ garlic cloves
- 1 avocado
- 1 lemon

Preparation

1. Book the broccoli and then toss in a pan with ½ tsp rapeseed oil.
2. Cook the chicken with the remaining oil and then slice each breast.
3. To make the pest, mix all the ingredients with a food processor. Set aside the basil for now.
4. Add the basil and lemon juice when the pesto is ready.
5. Serve the chicken breasts with broccoli, watercress and the avocado pesto in a large bowl.

Dinner: Green Juice** **(See page 24)

DAY 3

Breakfast: Green Juice (See page 24)

Lunch: Green Juice (See page 24)

Dinner: Kale and Red Onion Dhal with Buckwheat

Difficulty: Easy | Calories: 402 | Servings: 4

Fat: 7 g | Carbs: 71 g | Protein: 18 g

Ingredients

- 400 ml (14 oz.) coconut milk
- 100 g (3.5 oz.) kale
- 200 ml (7 oz.) water
- 160 g (5.6 oz.) buckwheat
- 160 g (5.6 oz.) lentils
- 2 tsp garam masala
- 3 tsp turmeric
- Grated ginger
- 1 tbsp olive oil
- 3 garlic cloves
- 1 red onion

Preparation

1. Cook the sliced onion in olive oil. Add the garlic, chilli (optional) and ginger and cook for a few minutes.
2. Add the spices (garam masala and turmeric) and a bit of water.
3. Cook for 1 more minute, then add the coconut milk, all the water and red lentils.
4. Stir well and cook for 20 minutes.
5. Add the kale and cook for a further 5 minutes.
6. Cook the buckwheat in boiling water. When ready, serve with the dhal.

DAY 4

Breakfast: Green Juice (See page 24)

Lunch: Green Juice (See page 24)

Dinner: Easy Spicy Rice

Difficulty: Easy | Calories: 269 | Servings: 6

Fat: 4 g | Carbs: 49 g | Protein: 7 g

Ingredients

- 100 g (3.5 oz.) peas
- 600 ml (21 oz.) hot chicken stock
- 300 g (10.5 oz.) long grain rice (or buckwheat)
- 1 tsp smoked paprika
- 1 tsp turmeric
- 1 small red pepper
- 1 small onion
- 1 tbsp olive oil
- ½ tsp chilli flakes
- Salt and pepper

Preparation

1. Cook the diced onion and red pepper in a saucepan for about 3 minutes.
2. Add the chilli flakes, smoked paprika and turmeric. Cook for another 2 minutes. Add a bit of water, if needed.
3. Add the chicken stock and rice. Season with salt and pepper. Leave to cook for 7-10 minutes.
4. Add the peas and stir well. Cover with a lid and leave to cook for 3 minutes.

DAY 5

Breakfast: Green Juice (See page 24)

Lunch: Green Juice (See page 24)

Dinner: Salmon Fishcakes

Difficulty: Medium | Calories: 329 | Servings: 4

Fat: 6 g | Carbs: 39 g | Protein: 27 g

Ingredients

- 1 kg (2.2 lbs) white potatoes
- 50 g (1.7 oz.) wholemeal flour
- 400 g (14.10 oz.) salmon
- 2 tbsp fresh parsley
- Salad to serve
- Salt and pepper
- Olive oil

Preparation

1. Place the potatoes in a pan, bring to the boil and cook until soft.
2. Meanwhile, rub the olive oil to coat your fish. Place it on a grill rack and cook for 3 minutes on each side.
3. Flake the fish once ready and add it to the potatoes.
4. Dress with lemon juice, salt and pepper, and add the parsley.
5. Shape your fishcake into 12 balls.
6. Roll each ball in the flour.
7. Preheat oven to 120 C (250 F).
8. Cook the fishcakes in oil for about 2 minutes, then put in the oven for a few more minutes.
9. Serve with your choice of salad.

DAY 6

Breakfast: Kale Omelette (See page 30)

Lunch: Green Juice (See page 24)

Dinner: Greek Style Lamb Kebabs

Difficulty: Medium | Calories: 455 | Servings: 4

Fat: 27 g | Carbs: 6 g | Protein: 46 g

Ingredients

- 8 skewers
- 900 g (31.7 oz.) lamb leg steaks
- 60 ml (2 oz.) olive oil
- 2 cloves garlic
- Salt and pepper
- The juice of 2 lemons

Preparation

1. Set the lamb aside and mix together all the ingredients.
2. Cut the lamb in cubes and leave it to marinate in the mixture for 2 hours.
3. Thread the lamb pieces onto the skewers and cook in your griddle pan or grill for 2-3 minutes on each side.
4. Serve with oregano or your choice of spices.

Day 7

Breakfast: Green Juice (See page 24)

Lunch: Yellow Split Pea and Spinach Dhal (See page 53)

Dinner: Roast Parsnips with Honey and Thyme

Difficulty: Easy | Calories: 134 | Servings: 8

Fat: 3 g | Carbs: 25 g | Protein: 1 g

Ingredients

- 6 medium parsnips
- 3 spring of thyme
- 2 tbsp runny honey
- 2 tbsp olive oil
- Salt and pepper

Preparation

1. Preheat oven to 220 C (400 F).
2. Place the parsnips in a roasting tray and season with olive oil, salt and pepper.
3. Scatter some thyme.
4. Roast for 20 minutes. Drizzle with honey and return to the oven for another 10 minutes.
5. Serve with additional thyme.

DAY 8

Breakfast: Green Juice *(See page 24)*

Lunch: Sweet Potato and Red Lentil Soup

Difficulty: Easy | Calories: 376 | Servings: 4

Fat: 8 g | Carbs: 61 g | Protein: 15 g

Ingredients

- 200 g (7 oz.) red lentils
- 1 onion
- 3 medium carrots
- 2 bell peppers
- 2 cloves garlic
- 2 litres (70 oz.) vegetable stock
- 2 small parsnips
- 1 medium sweet potato
- 1 tsp dried chilli flakes
- Salt and pepper

Preparation

1. Fry the onions in olive oil for 5 minutes.
2. Add the carrots, parsnips, peppers, and sweet potato, and fry for a few more minutes. Add the garlic ginger and chilli.
3. Add the vegetable stock and the lentils. Season with salt and pepper and bring to the boil. Cook for 20 minutes.
4. blend the soup with a food processor and serve with buckwheat or your choice of salad.

Dinner: Spinach Style Red Wine, Borlotti Bean and Lamb Shank Casserole *(See page 59)*

DAY 9

Breakfast: Green Juice (See page 24)

Lunch: Cider, Cream and Mustard Pork (See page 53)

Dinner: Baked Potatoes with Spicy Chickpea Stew

Difficulty: Medium | Calories: 500 | Servings: 6

Fat: 10 g | Carbs: 91 g | Protein: 19 g

Ingredients

- 2 x 400 g (28 oz.) tins chopped tomatoes
- 2 yellow peppers
- 2 x 400 g (28 oz.) tins chickpeas
- 4 cloves garlic
- 2 red onions
- 6 baking potatoes
- 2 tbsp parsley
- 2 tbsp turmeric
- 2 tbsp cumin seeds
- Grated ginger
- 2 tbsp parsley
- 2 tbsp unsweetened cocoa powder
- Water
- Salt and pepper

Preparation

1. Preheat the oven to 220 C (400 F).
2. Bake the baking potatoes for 1 hour.
3. Meanwhile, cook the chopped onion in olive oil for about 5 minutes.
4. Add the ginger, cumin, garlic and chilli (optional). Cook for 1 minute, then add the turmeric and a bit of water.
5. After a few minutes, add the cocoa powder, chickpeas (including their water), tomatoes and yellow pepper. Bring to the boil and leave to simmer for 45 minutes. You must get a thick sauce.
6. Add the parsley and season with salt and pepper.
7. Serve the stew on top of your baked potatoes.

DAY 10

Breakfast: Green Juice (See page 24)

Lunch: Easy Chicken Curry

Difficulty: Easy | Calories: 472 | Servings: 4

Fat: 13 g | Carbs: 54 g | Protein: 37 g

Ingredients

- 8 boneless, skinless chicken thighs
- 400 ml (14 oz.) coconut milk
- 200 g (7 oz.) buckwheat
- 2 tbsp fresh coriander
- 2 tsp garam masala
- 2 tsp ground turmeric
- 2 tsp ground cumin
- Fresh ginger
- 3 garlic cloves
- 1 red onion
- 1 cinnamon stick
- 6 cardamom pods
- Olive oil

Preparation

1. Place the ginger, onion and garlic in a food processor to make a paste.
2. Add the cumin, turmeric and garam masala and stir together.
3. Cook the chopped chicken thighs in olive oil and, after a few minutes, add the curry paste.
4. After 2-3 minutes, add half the coconut milk, cardamom and cinnamon. Allow to simmer for ½ hour.
5. Cook the buckwheat while the chicken curry is cooking.
6. Add some fresh coriander and serve everything together.

Dinner: Pasta with Spinach and Blue Cheese Sauce ***(See page 44)***

DAY 11

Breakfast: Turmeric Pancakes

Difficulty: Easy | Calories: 329 | Servings: 4
Fat: 11 g | Carbs: 45 g | Protein: 11 g

Ingredients

- 200 g (7 oz.) self-rising flour
- 200 ml (7 oz.) soy milk
- 25 g butter
- 3 eggs
- 2 tbsp honey
- 1 tsp baking powder
- ½ tsp ground turmeric
- ¼ tsp ground ginger

Preparation

1. Mix all the ingredients in a bowl and whisk well.
2. Add the butter in a large non-stick frying pan.
3. Add 2 tbsp batter for each pancake and cook for 2-3 minutes on both sides.
4. Serve with lemon curd, fresh fruits and ginger.

Lunch: Roast Beef Curry (See page 57)

Dinner: One-Pot Harissa Chicken and Butternut Squash Pilaf (See page 50)

DAY 12

Breakfast: Kale Omelette *(See page 30)*

Lunch: Green Juice Salad

Difficulty: Easy | Calories: 290 | Servings: 1

Fat: 23 g | Carbs: 21 g | Protein: 6 g

Ingredients

- 6 walnuts halves
- 2 celery sticks
- Some fresh rocket
- Grated ginger
- The juice of ½ lemon
- Fresh kale
- Parsley
- ½ green apple
- 1 tbsp olive oil
- Salt and pepper

Preparation

1. Squeeze the lemon juice and mix it with the ginger and olive oil. Season with salt and pepper and stir well.
2. Place the kale in a serving bowl and leave to marinate with the lemon juice dressing.
3. After a few minutes, add all the other ingredients and mix well.

Dinner: Lamb Jalfrezi *(See page 55)*

DAY 13

Breakfast: Green Juice *(See page 24)*

Lunch: Pasta with Spinach and Blue Cheese Sauce *(See page 44)*

Dinner: Kale Salad with Lemon Tahini Dressing

Difficulty: Easy | Calories: 274 | Servings: 2

Fat: 21 g | Carbs: 10 g | Protein: 10 g

Ingredients

- 50 g (1.7 oz.) tahini
- 200 g (7 oz.) kale
- 1 tbsp olive oil
- 1 garlic clove
- The juice of 1 lemon

Preparation

1. You can start by making the dressing. Mix the tahini, lemon juice and garlic with a little bit of cold water in a small bowl.
2. Stir fry the kale for a couple of minutes in oil.
3. Add half the dressing and cook for another minute.
4. Transfer to a serving plate and add the remaining dressing.

DAY 14

Breakfast: Green Juice (See page 24)

Lunch: Soy Salmon & Broccoli Traybake

Difficulty: Medium | Calories: 310 | Servings: 4

Fat: 17 g | Carbs: 3 g | Protein: 35 g

Ingredients

- 4 salmon fillets
- 2 tbsp soy sauce
- The juice of ½ lemon
- ½ lemon
- Fresh spring onions
- 1 head broccoli florets

Preparation

1. Heat oven to 180 C (350 F).
2. Arrange the broccoli florets and the salmon fillets in a baking tray.
3. Season with lemon juice and add the lemon sliced into quarters.
4. Drizzle with olive oil and top with the spring onions.
5. Bake for 15 minutes.
6. Sprinkle with soy sauce and return to the oven for 5 more minutes.
7. Sprinkle with additional spring onions before serving.

Dinner: Spinach Style Red Wine, Borlotti Bean and Lamb Shank Casserole (See page 59)

DAY 15

Breakfast: Date & Walnut Cinnamon Bites

Difficulty: Easy | Calories: 168 | Servings: 1

Fat: 8 g | Carbs: 21 g | Protein: 2 g

Ingredients

- 3 pitted Medjool dates
- 3 walnut halves
- Ground cinnamon

Preparation

1. Cut each walnut half into slices.
2. Repeat the same process with the dates.
3. Place a slice of walnut on top of each date slice.
4. Season with cinnamon and serve.

Lunch: Easy One-Pot Vegan Paella (See page 31)

Dinner: Buckwheat and Beetroot Salad (See page 48)

DAY 16

Breakfast: Green Juice (See page 24)

Lunch: Cider, Cream and Mustard Pork (See page 52)

Dinner: Strawberry, Tomato & Watercress Salad with Pink Pepper Dressing

Difficulty: Easy | Calories: 128 | Servings: 4

Fat: 9 g | Carbs: 8 g | Protein: 2 g

Ingredients

- 300 g (10.5 oz.) strawberries
- 100 g (3.5 oz.) watercress
- 250 g (8.8 oz.) mixed tomatoes

Dressing

- 3 tbsp extra virgin olive oil
- 30 g (1 oz.) strawberries
- ½ tbsp lemon
- 1 tbsp pink peppercorns
- ½ tbsp honey

Preparation

1. Fry the peppercorns for a couple of minutes.
2. With a pestle and mortar, process the peppercorn with salt and the strawberries. Smash all ingredients to a paste.
3. For the salad, stir in the lemon juice and honey. Whisk the dressing with the olive oil.
4. Assemble the salad with the strawberries, cut into slices, chopped tomatoes and the watercress.

DAY 17

Breakfast: Green Juice *(See page 24)*

Lunch: Broccoli & Kale Green Soup

Difficulty: Easy | Calories: 182 | Servings: 2

Fat: 8 g | Carbs: 14 g | Protein: 10 g

Ingredients

- 500 ml (17.6 oz.) vegetable stock
- 1 tbsp sunflower oil
- ½ tsp ground coriander
- 2 garlic cloves
- 1 piece fresh turmeric root
- 200 g (7 oz.) courgettes
- 100 g (3.5 oz.) kale
- 85 g (2.9 oz.) broccoli
- 1 lime
- Fresh parsley

Preparation

1. Fry the garlic, coriander, ginger and turmeric in a deep pan with the oil. Add 3 tbsp water to get a thicker texture.
2. Add the courgette and the part of the stock, and leave to simmer for a few minutes.
3. Add kale, broccoli and lime juice. Add the rest of the stock and leave to cook until the vegetables are ready.
4. Pour everything in a blender with chopped parsley and process until smooth.
5. Season with salt, lime zest and more parsley.

Dinner: Pork Stroganoff (See page 61)

DAY 18

Breakfast: Kale Omelette (See page 30)

Lunch: Lamb Jalfrezi (See page 55)

Dinner: Salmon Salad

Difficulty: Easy | Calories: 350 | Servings: 2

Fat: 10 g | Carbs: 30 g | Protein: 30 g

Ingredients

- 2 salmon fillets
- 100 g (3.5 oz.) couscous
- 30 g (1 oz.) watercress
- 200 g (7 oz.) broccoli
- 1 tbsp olive oil
- Pumpkin seeds
- Pomegranate seeds
- The juice of 1 lemon
- Lemon wedges

Preparation

1. Pour boiling water over the couscous and season with olive oil.
2. Cook the salmon and broccoli in the steam for 3 minutes.
3. Meanwhile, mix the lemon juice with remaining oil.
4. Sprinkle all the seeds over the broccoli and season the couscous with the lemon dressing.
5. Add some chopped watercress and lemon wedges before serving.

DAY 19

Breakfast: Green Juice *(See page 24)*

Lunch: Pasta with Spinach and Blue Cheese Sauce *(See page 44)*

Dinner: Malabar Prawns

Difficulty: Medium | Calories: 171 | Servings: 4

Fat: 8 g | Carbs: 4 g | Protein: 19 g

Ingredients

- 400 g (14 oz.) king prawns
- 40 g (1.4 oz.) ginger
- 4 tsp Kashmiri chilli powder
- 2 tsp turmeric
- 1 tbsp vegetable oil
- 4 tsp lemon juice
- 4 curry leaves
- 1 onion
- 40 g (1.4 oz.) fresh coconut
- Coriander leaves
- Black pepper

Preparation

1. Toss the prawns with the chilli powder, lemon juice, turmeric and grated ginger. Set aside
2. Fry the curry leaves, sliced ginger, onion and chilli with the oil. Cook for 10 minutes, then add the black pepper.
3. Add the prawns and cook for about 2 minutes.
4. Season with lemon juice, coriander leaves and coconut.

DAY 20

Breakfast: Green Juice (See page 24)

Lunch: Chicken, Kale & Sprout Stir-Fry

Difficulty: Medium | Calories: 390 | Servings: 2

Fat: 6 g | Carbs: 45 g | Protein: 35 g

Ingredients

- 100 g (3.5 oz.) soba noodle
- 25 g (0.9 oz.) fresh ginger
- 100 g (3.5 oz.) Brussels sprout
- 2 chicken breasts
- 100 g (3.5 oz.) shredded curly kale
- 1 red pepper
- 2 tsp sesame oil
- 1 tbsp soy sauce
- 2 tbsp white wine vinegar
- The juice of 1 lime

Preparation

1. Cook the noodles and set aside.
2. Cook the kale for a couple of minutes.
3. Add half the oil and the chicken and cook until ready.
4. In the remaining oil, fry the pepper, sprouts and the ginger.
5. Return the meat and kale, and add the noodles.
6. Mix a bit of water with the vinegar, soy sauce and lime juice to create a sauce.
7. Serve all ingredients together.

Dinner: Roast Beef Curry ***(See page 57)***

DAY 21

Breakfast: Kale Omelette *(See page 30)*

Lunch: Cider, Cream and Mustard Pork *(See page 52)*

Dinner: Turmeric Baked Salmon

Difficulty: Medium | Calories: 490 | Servings: 1

Fat: 18 g | Carbs: 31 g | Protein: 29 g

Ingredients

- 200 g (7 oz.) skinned salmon
- 40 g (1.2 oz.) red onion
- 60 g (2 oz.) tinned green lentils
- 150 g (5.3 oz.) celery
- 1 tsp mild curry powder
- 2 tsp extra virgin olive oil
- 1 tsp ground turmeric
- 130 g (4.5 oz.) tomato (cut into wedges)
- 100 ml (3.5 oz.) vegetable stock
- 1 garlic clove
- Chopped parsley

Preparation

1. Heat the oven to 200 C (400 F).
2. Fry the garlic, onion, chilli, celery and ginger in olive oil. Add the curry powder and cook for a few minutes.
3. Add the stock, lentils and tomatoes and leave to simmer for 10 minutes.
4. Meanwhile, mix the oil, lemon juice and turmeric in a bowl. Rub the mixture over the salmon.
5. Bake the salmon for 10 minutes.
6. Serve with celery and parsley.

DAY 22

Breakfast: Mushroom Scramble Eggs

Difficulty: Easy | Calories: 190 | Servings: 1
Fat: 8 g | Carbs: 21 g | Protein: 2 g

Ingredients

- 2 eggs
- 20 g (0.7 g) kale
- 5 g (0.17 oz.) parsley
- A handful of button mushrooms (thinly sliced)
- 1 tsp mild curry powder
- 1 tsp ground turmeric
- 1 tsp extra virgin olive oil

Preparation

1. Mix the curry and turmeric powder with a bit of water until you get a light paste.
2. Steam the kale.
3. Cook the mushrooms in a frying pan with the olive oil.
4. Add the eggs and the curry paste.
5. Sprinkle with parsley before serving.

Lunch: Buckwheat with Mushrooms Salad (See page 33)

Dinner: Goat Cheese Salad with Walnut Dressing (See page 35)

DAY 23

Breakfast: Date and Walnut Porridge

Difficulty: easy | Calories: 150 | Servings: 1

Fat: 7 g | Carbs: 2 g | Protein: 31 g

Ingredients

- 200 ml (7 oz.) soy milk
- 35 g (1.2 oz.) Buckwheat flakes
- 50 g (1.7 oz.) fresh strawberries
- 1 Medjool date
- 1 tsp walnut butter

Preparation

1. Pour the milk in a pan and heat gently. Add the date and cook for 1 minute.
2. Add the buckwheat flakes and cook until you get a porridge-like consistency.
3. Stir in the walnut butter and add fresh strawberries.

Lunch: Spinach Style Red Wine, Borlotti Bean and Lamb Shank Casserole ***(See page 59)***

Dinner: Cashew Buckwheat Curry with Garlic Kale ***(See page 36)***

DAY 24

Breakfast: Kale Omelette (See page 30)

Lunch: Sirtfood Shakshuka

Difficulty: Medium | Calories: 301 | Servings: 1

Fat: 16 g | Carbs: 12 g | Protein: 31 g

Ingredients

- 40 g (1.4 oz.) red onion
- 30 g (1 oz.) celery
- 400 g (14.1 oz.) chopped tomatoes
- 30 g (1 oz.) kale
- 1 tsp extra virgin olive oil
- 1 garlic clove
- 2 medium eggs
- 1 tsp ground cumin
- 1 tsp paprika
- 1 tsp ground turmeric
- 1 tbsp chopped parsley
- 1 bird's eye chilli

Preparation

1. Fry the garlic, celery, chilli, onion and spices for 2 minutes.
2. Add the tomatoes and leave to simmer for 20 minutes.
3. Add the kale and, when the sauce is thick enough, stir in the parsley.
4. Make some space in the sauce and crack the eggs into them. Leave them to cook for 10 minutes.

Dinner: Cheesy Buckwheat with Kale and Mushrooms (See page 46)

DAY 25

Breakfast: Mushroom Scramble Eggs

Difficulty: Easy | Calories: 109 | Servings: 1

Fat: 6 g | Carbs: 12 g | Protein: 3 g

Ingredients

- 1 large egg
- ¼ tsp baking soda
- 1 ½ tsp baking powder
- ½ cup unsweetened cocoa powder
- ¼ cup melted coconut oil
- ¼ tsp almond extract
- 1 ½ cups unsweetened almond milk
- ½ tsp vanilla extract
- 2 tbsp honey
- 1 cup buckwheat flour

Preparation

1. Whisk the cocoa powder, baking powder, baking soda and buckwheat flour in a bowl. Season with salt.
2. In another bowl, mix the almond milk, vanilla and almond extract, coconut oil and the egg.
3. Mix the wet ingredients with the dry ones.
4. Spray a large non-stick skillet with olive oil.
5. Pour a handful of mixture for each pancake into the skillet.
6. Cook for a couple of minutes on both sides.
7. Serve with your choice of toppings.

Lunch: Easy One-Pot Vegan Paella (See page 31)

Dinner: Pork Stroganoff (See page 61)

DAY 26

Breakfast: Green Juice (See page 24)

Lunch: Turkey Tikka Masala Meatballs with Bombay new Potatoes (with Raw Courgette Salad) (See page 63)

Dinner: Italian Kale Salad

Difficulty: Easy | Calories: 50 | Servings: 4

Fat: 4 g | Carbs: 1 g | Protein: 1 g

Ingredients

- 300 g (10.5 oz.) kale
- 3 tbsp red wine vinegar
- 3 tbsp olive oil
- 3 garlic cloves

Preparation

1. Cook the kale in a large pan with oil, garlic and vinegar.
2. Once cooked, season with salt.
3. Serve with your choice of meat or buckwheat rice.

DAY 27

Breakfast: Green Juice *(See page 24)*

Lunch: Red Chicory, Pear & Hazelnut Salad

Difficulty: Easy | Calories: 176 | Servings: 4

Fat: 15 g | Carbs: 8 g | Protein: 2 g

Ingredients

- 25 g (0.8 oz.) toasted hazelnut
- 2 heads of red chicory
- Rocket leaves
- 2 ripe red Williams pears

Dressing

- 2 tbsp olive oil
- 1 tsp cider vinegar
- 1 tsp green peppercorns in brine
- 2 tbsp sunflower oil

Preparation

1. Mix all the dressing ingredients and set aside.
2. Discard the chicory stalk ends and the outer leaves.
3. Separate the remaining leaves and arrange on a plate.
4. Quarter each pear lengthways.
5. Arrange pear slices on top of the chicory leaves and season with the dressing and some rocket leaves.

Dinner: One-Pot Harissa Chicken and Butternut Squash Pilaf ***(See page 50)***

DAY 28

Breakfast: Kale Omelette (See page 30)

Lunch: Yellow Split Pea and Spinach Dhal (See page 53)

Dinner: Sirtfood Chicken & Kale Curry

Difficulty: Medium | Calories: 313 | Servings: 4

Fat: 21 g | Carbs: 9 g | Protein: 21 g

Ingredients

- 400 g (14 oz.) skinless and boneless chicken thighs
- 200 ml (7 oz.) coconut milk
- 500 ml (17.6 oz.) boiling water
- 2 red onions
- 175 g (6.2 oz.) chopped tomatoes
- 1 chicken stockpot
- 1 tbsp curry powder
- 1 tbsp freshly chopped ginger
- 3 garlic cloves
- 1 tbsp olive oil
- 2 tbsp ground turmeric
- 2 cardamom pods
- 2 birds eye chilli

Preparation

1. Allow the chicken to marinate for ½ hour in 1 tsp of oil and 1 tbsp of turmeric.
2. Fry the chicken and then set aside.
3. Cook the garlic, chilli, ginger and onion in the remaining oil.
4. Add 1 tbsp turmeric and the curry powder and cook for a couple of minutes.
5. Add coconut milk, chicken stock, tomatoes and cardamom pods. Leave to simmer for ½ hour.
6. Add the chicken back to the reduced sauce and add the kale. Cook until the meat is ready.
7. Serve with chopped coriander and buckwheat rice.

Printed in Great Britain
by Amazon